Aromatherapy & Essential Oil Recipes for Beginners

ALICIA WATTERS

Use Proven Aromatherapy & Essential Oils to Improve your Health, Skin, Hair, and to Lose Weight.

2nd Edition

Aromatherapy & Essential Oil Recipes For Beginners 2nd Edition

Copyright 2014 by Alicia Watters - All rights reserved.

Table Of Contents

Introduction

I want to thank you and congratulate you for purchasing the book, *Aromatherapy & Essential Oil Recipes for Beginners: Use Proven Aromatherapy & Essential Oils to Improve your Health, Skin, Hair, and to Lose Weight.*

This book contains proven steps and strategies on how to use basic essential oil formulas for various health concerns.

Also included are useful information about aromatherapy, essential oils, and blending basics to help you go through your aromatherapy experience safely and successfully.

Thanks again for purchasing this book, I hope you enjoy it!

Chapter 1 – Basic Information about Aromatherapy and Essential Oils

Although the practice was only named *aromatherapy* in the 20th century, the use of aromatic plants for health has been around since ancient times. Truth be told, mankind has been relying on the application of essential oils for a variety of purposes (e.g., as a beauty aid or as a medical treatment for thousands of years), and the practice actually has roots in the burning of roots, leaves, and tree gums as far back as when man first discovered fire.

Aromatherapy initially began with the use of incense, when the burned parts of the plants filled the air with perfumed smoke. Legend also has it that the modern word "perfume" was actually derived from the Latin word *per fumum*, which literally translates into "through smoke."

It wasn't until around 7000 to 4000 B.C.E., however, that early man discovered that the application of heated animal fats to aromatic plants led to the former absorbing the aromatic and medicinal properties of the latter. Upon the discovery of such, early man eventually came to apply the concoction on their skin either as a beauty treatment or as a more tangible way to use scented fats to uplift or revitalize their moods.

It wasn't long before civilized men derived another product from scented plants; this time in the form of aromatic water (the precursor to the modern-day cologne or perfume). The first perfume recipes combined aromatic, essential oils with water and alcohol to produce a concoction that was applied to the face and hair for cosmetic purposes and was also ingested as a form of medicinal treatment.

Aromatherapy & Essential Oil Recipes For Beginners 2nd Edition

As human civilizations became more stable and prosperous, they eventually resorted to combining the different forms of aromatherapy into blends that were meant to provide holistic healing for the human body.

The Chinese culture may have been the first to perform such practices, but it was the Egyptians who first used aromatic plants and incenses. The ancient Egyptians also used to burn incenses made out of aromatic wood material, spices, and herbs originally for religious purposes. They also used oils after baths since they knew about its moisturizing effects on the skin. The invention of the rudimentary distillation method and apparatus is also commonly ascribed to the ancient Egyptians, which they used to generate scented oils derived from various herbs and plants to be used in religious rituals and beauty regimens alike.

A few centuries later, the ancient Greeks also came to adapt the craft and practice of aromatherapy. Hippocrates, the legendary "Father of Modern Medicine," was among the advocates of using aromatherapy as a form of medical treatment and was among the first ancient Greek physicians to study the effects of aromatic oils on one's mood, health, and overall well-being.

But the real origins of aromatherapy's breakthrough into the medical world lay in a rather dramatic story from the nineteenth century. It all started when a French chemist by the name of Rene-Maurice Gatttefosse sustained a bad burn while he was at work in his laboratory. Smarting from the pain, he impulsively plunged his hand into the nearest vat of liquid, which happened to contain lavender essential oils. Not only did the fragrance of the lavender oil soothe his frazzled nerves, but his burn healed quickly afterward without a scar. With his interest in the medical possibilities of essential oils piqued, he eventually embarked on a study of the medicinal qualities of each essential oil and ended up coining the very term "aromatherapy." Gatttefosse's labors culminated in the ultimate aromatherapy reference, a book he called "Aromatherapie: Les Huiles Essentielles Hormones Vegetales," loosely translated into the English language as "Gatttefosse's Aromatherapy." The book was so instrumental to the progress of aromatherapy that it's still widely used among physicians and aromatherapy enthusiasts today.

Gatttefosse's foray into the world of aromatherapy would inspire others to follow suit, leading to some significant developments in the field. Aromatherapy was eventually used by the French physician Dr. Jean Valnet to treat soldiers suffering from flesh wounds and burns during World War II. He would eventually go on to write a book on the subject called "The Practice of Aromatherapy." The Austrian biochemist, Madame Marguerite Maury, on the other hand, pioneered the use of aromatherapy in cosmetic products. She would later incorporate aromatic oils into the practice of massage.

Today, aromatherapy or otherwise known as *essential oils therapy* is used to treat various health concerns such as stress, weight loss, skin health, and more. In this practice, the essential oils are extracted from a plant's leaves, flowers, bark, rind, roots, or stalks. After this process, the extracts are mixed together with oil, alcohol, or lotion so they can be applied on a person's skin directly, sprayed, or inhaled. These aromatic oils are also used for massage and for baths.

Since aromatherapy uses a lot of natural medicinal ingredients, it is regarded by researchers as a completely safe and effective treatment practice. Basically, the kind of oils used to treat certain ailments contains ingredients which are proven by science to have substantiated effects in treating the symptoms.

Other than parts of volatile plants, modern aromatherapy also uses other natural ingredients such as *jojoba, milk powders, hydrosols, herbs, sea salts, sugars, clays,* and *muds.* Although some products that contain synthetic materials are looked down upon by modern holistic aromatherapy, they are still available in the market with debatable efficacy.

The Benefits of Aromatherapy

Since ancient times, humans have been attracted to natural fragrant aromas. During ancient Egyptian festivals, women wore fragrant *cones* on their heads that would melt in the sun; releasing their pleasant smell.

When inhaled, the natural oils used in aromatherapy triggers a psychological as well as a physical effect on a person. The fragrance is known to produce either sedative or stimulating effects on a person's brain, as well as the healing properties of the ingredients used. The essential oils also apply their therapeutic benefits once the naturally occurring chemicals in the materials used are introduced to the person's lungs. Some of the more specific health benefits posed by the inhalation of essential oils include the following:

1.) Pain management and relief. The inhalation of certain aromatic oils can actually help lessen the sort of pain that comes with some common ailments. A blend of eucalyptus and peppermint essential oils, for instance, can relieve headaches when inhaled. Clary sage oils are also great pain relievers, and have been commonly prescribed as an alternative to pain medications that target dysmenorrheal or menstrual cramps.

2.) Blood pressure regulation. Tense patients who suffer from high blood pressure can find relief in inhaling certain essential oils that relax the body enough to let one's blood pressure drop to safer levels.

3.)   Mood relief. Individuals who suffer from anxiety disorders or depression can find a sense of relief in inhaling the aromas of essential oils derived from citrus fruits or from other plants that are known for their bright, vibrant fragrances. Getting a massage while lighting a burner containing lemon, orange, or verbena essential oils can actually do wonders for boosting one's despondent state of mind.

4.)   Stress relief. This health benefit is perhaps the one that is most associated with aromatherapy, given that spas and clinics that use essential oils often aim to bring down one's stress levels. Lavender and chamomile essential oils, for instance, are often prescribed to soothe frazzled nerves and to aid in bringing about untroubled sleep.

When applied directly to the skin, the essential oils used in aromatherapy produces a variety of therapeutic benefits. Some essential oils contain antibacterial properties to help promote the healing and prevention of superficial skin wounds and disorders such as *staph infection* and *acne*. Other essential oils (especially those used for massage therapies) relieves numerous aches and pains in a person's physical body. The application of peppermint or eucalyptus essential oils, for instance, have been known to soothe tired or overworked muscles and can also relieve minor to moderate headaches.

Other physical benefits of the use of essential oils include the treatment of hormonal imbalances, metabolism conditions, fatigue, the promotion of deep sleep and relaxation. Certain essential oils are also proven to be effective in treating harmful bacteria such as *Escherichia coli, salmonella typhimurium, listeria monocytogenes,* and *staphylococcus aureus.*

There are also scientifically-validated psychological benefits of essential oils including the most common *boost in overall state of well-being, calming effect,* and *stress relief.* Essential oils are also proven to produce positive results in treating anxiety, depression, and even age-related mental conditions such as *Alzheimer's disease.* The use of certain essential oils is also suggested by clinical tests to boost short term memory, which is a relevant factor in the quality of a person's long term memory.

Some essential oils, such as sweet almond oil, are also applied as effective beauty aids. Apart from its superior moisturizing quality, sweet almond oils have also been known to prevent or treat stretch marks.

When applied to the skin, tea tree essential oils, on the other hand, can treat and prevent acne. The cooling effect of the said essential oil has also been known to alleviate skin redness and irritation, and can also minimize swelling brought about by skin pustules or eruptions. (It should be noted, however, that essential oils should never be applied to broken skin or open wounds as this could lead to infections.)

Should I purchase or create my own essential oils?

Blending your own essential oils is possible, but requires time, knowledge, and some money. The main advantage of creating your own supply of essential oils is that you are 100% sure that you used natural ingredients, which is one of the defining factors that determine the quality and effectiveness of the product. However, creating homemade essential oils may be too time-consuming, so it is recommended for beginners to purchase your supply of essential oils. Before purchasing essential oils, take note of the following basic guidelines.

1. **Look for "100% essential oil" in labels.** Products diluted at around 3-5% in base oil are relatively cheaper, but may not have the same potency as 100% essential oils. These 100% essential oils are also referred to as *Undiluted* or *Unadulterated* essential oils. However, this does not imply that 100% pure essential oils are the only *real* products and the rest are useless imitations. Diluted oils still have their own uses (especially for direct skin applications), so it's better to perform a little research about the product and its uses.

2. **Test the fragrance of every essential oil you buy.** Products that produce relatively weak aromas are most likely of poor quality, especially if you are shopping at independent distributors. Well-extracted essential oils can easily be detected basing on the subtlety and the richness of its fragrance. In other words, higher quality essential oils usually smell stronger. When in doubt, you can purchase only samples from these suppliers.

3. **Find the botanical names in the essential oils before you purchase.** Botanical names are actually *Latin names* given to species of plants and flowers. Looking for these names in the bottles of essential oil products is important. There are safety issues of using products whose ingredients are not listed with accurate botanical names.

4. **Check the company supplying the essential oil.** Given that the market is flooded with cheap and diluted bottles of essential oils, do make sure that you purchase yours from a reliable supplier. Certain things that make a good essential oil supplier include the following:

a. **They are a small, preferably homegrown company that cultivates a relationship with the distillers of their oils (unless the company distills the oils themselves).** Large conglomerates often don't specialize in the manufacturing and bottling of essential oils (due to the relatively low profit margins it brings), so you may not be getting a quality product if you purchase a bottle of essential oil from a generic brand owned by such. Also, smaller and localized companies usually focus on deriving essential oils from the herbs and plants that are indigenous to the area, making their products more effective, authentic, as well more environment-friendly.

b. **They can readily provide you with material safety data sheets upon request.** These normally involve the sorts of herbs and/or plants included in their essential oil blends. A reputable supplier should have undergone the proper research prior and should also be updated with the latest news in the aromatherapy field, and should thus be able to satisfactorily answer or address any safety concerns with regards to their product.

c. **They are established in the field of aromatherapy and enjoy a largely uncontroversial reputation.** Companies that achieve that sort of status get there by following safe practices and adhering to the right food and beverage safety standards. Beware of unheard-of and possibly bogus companies that peddle essential oils at suspiciously low prices.

d. **The supply company is owned by an aromatherapy or essential oil specialist and**

practitioner. It often takes years of study to become such, and only such individuals are fully qualified to dispense advice about the proper usage of aromatherapy oils.

5. **Look at how the essential oils are bottled or stored.** Since essential oils are vulnerable to heat or sunlight (the warmth can cause their aroma to dissipate), they should be stored in either dark, opaque-colored glass bottles or in stainless steel containers. Thus, you shouldn't buy from suppliers who store their aromatic oils differently (especially those who sell oils packaged in clear, flimsy plastic bottles), or from those who store their products by the window, directly in front of the sun.

6. **Given the choice, opt for bottles of essential oils with dripolator plugs rather than the traditional eyedroppers.** Dripolators are superior to traditional eyedroppers in evenly distributing minute amounts of essential oils, and are also better at preventing the bottle's contents from spilling even when the cap is removed.

Chapter 2 – About Essential Oils

Essential oils extracted from the leaves, bark, roots, or other parts of a plant are distilled usually by steam or water. The extracted essential oils contain the concentrated therapeutic properties of the plant while in a liquid form that can be easily used for various applications. They are also quite volatile, prone to evaporating quickly if left exposed in an open space for a while. Essential oils can also be blended with other oils or *carrier oils* such as sweet almond oil, and grapeseed oil, but may produce slightly varied effects rather than the main therapeutic benefit of the original plant.

Aromatic oils are usually derived from tiny sacs or gobbets within the fruit, and are derived through a variety of methods, which can include one or two of the following:

1.) Steam distillation. This is the most common method of distilling essential oils, and generally involves bubbling steam through a plant's insides, which causes them to vaporize at a lower temperature. Since the steam used in this distillation technique is gentler than using outright heat, it's especially ideal for heat-sensitive plants.

2.) Cold pressing. Also called expression, this method applies no heat whatsoever and instead relies on a significantly high amount of mechanical pressure to extract the highly fragrant oils from fruit peels.

Safety

Aromatherapy essential oil products are generally safe, but one must use them only with reliable knowledge. This doesn't imply that you shouldn't use pure essential oil products with confidence as a beginner. However, to avoid any undesired effects related to the improper use of essential oils, take note of the following safety guidelines:

1. **On-skin applications** – Keep in mind that unadulterated or undiluted essential oils are highly concentrated, and are therefore highly potent. This means that the applications of essential oils must be administered with great care. As a basic rule, avoid using undiluted essential oils directly on the skin, especially on sensitive areas such as the mouth or around the eyes. However, there are certain unadulterated essential oils that are safe for on-skin use such as *lavender* and *tea tree oil,* but it still depends on the skin sensitivity of the user.

2. **Allergic reactions** – Given that aromatherapy essential oils are produced with a wide range of natural ingredients; there are few individuals who may be allergic to some products. As a rule of thumb, always test 1-2 drops of the undiluted essential oil on a small part of your skin. Cover the area with a bandage and avoid getting the area wet for at least 24 hours. If you experience no discomfort or allergic reactions, then the product can be safely used.

3. **Maximum usage** – Essential oils are highly concentrated and very potent, so avoid using too much of the product. Always follow application instructions at all times with constant vigilance.

4. **Be aware of hazardous oils** – Remember that there are specific essential oils that can only be used by professional aromatherapy practitioners. Here is the list of essential oils that should never be used in aromatherapy by beginners:

   a. **Arnica** *(Arnica Montana)*

b. **Almond, Bitter** *(Prunus Dulcis var. Amara)*

c. **Ajowan** *(Trachyspermum Copticum)*

d. **Boldo Leaf** *(Peumus boldus)*

e. **Birch, Sweet** *(Betula Lenta)*

f. **Broom, Spanish** *(Spartium Junceum)*

g. **Buchu (Barosma betulina)**

h. **Camphor, Yellow** *(Cinnamomum Camphora)*

i. **Camphor, Brown** *(Cinnamomum Camphora)*

j. **Calamus** *(Acorus Calamus var. Angustatus)*

k. **Cascarilla** *(Croton Eluteria)*

l. **Chervil** *(Anthriscus Cerefolium)*

m. **Deertongue** *(Carphephorus Odoratissimus)*

n. **Garlic** *(Allium Sativum)*

o. **Horseradish** *(Armoracia Rusticana)*

p. **Jaborandi** *(Pilocarpus Jaborandi)*

q. **Melilotus** *(Melilotus Officinalis)*

r. **Mustard** *(Brassica Nigra)*

s. **Mugwort** *(Artemisia Vulgaris)*

t. **Narcissus** *(Narcissus poeticus)*

u. **Nutmeg** *(Myristica fragrans)*

v. **Onion** *(Allium Cepa)*

w. **Parsley** *(Petroselinum sativum, carum sativum)*

x. ***Pennyroyal*** *(Mentha Pulegium)*

y. ***Rue*** *(Ruta Graveolens)*

z. ***Sassafras*** *(Sassafras Albidum)*

aa.   ***Tansy*** *(Tanacetum vulgare) this one is also known to induce miscarriages in pregnant women.*

bb.   ***Tonka*** *(Dipteryx odorata)*

cc.   ***Thuja*** *(Thuja Occidentalis)*

dd.   ***Turmeric*** *(Curcuma longa)*

ee.   ***Wormseed*** *(Chenopodium Ambrosioides var. Anthelminticum)*

ff. ***Wormwood*** *(Artemisia Absinthium)*

gg.   ***Wintergreen*** *(Gaultheria Procumbens)*

5. **Fire hazard** – Keep in mind that essential oils are flammable liquids. For safety, store your supply of essential oils away from objects that may cause accidental ignitions such as lighters or stoves.

6. **Keep them away from children** – Fragrance is one of the essential oils' defining qualities. With this being said, there are certain essential oil products such as *citrus oils* that may smell inviting to drink. It is important that essential oils should be handled only by adults to avoid poisoning.

7. **Be especially careful when applying essential oils that can cause your skin to become very sensitive to light.** Citrus oils are particularly prone to irritating skin and to making it more vulnerable to light exposure, whether it's the sun or from a more artificial light source. Bergamot essential oils, in particular,

contain a photosensitizer called bergaptene that causes the skin to develop dark, uneven patches under sunlight or harsh lighting. (Although you can also purchase especially-formulated bergaptene-free bergamot essential oils.) If you really must apply citrus oils to your skin, it would be better to do so at night or indoors, where one is less exposed to harsh lighting or sunlight. In case this is not possible, you should wait for about four hours after applying the essential oil prior to heading out into the sunlight.

Other essential oils that are known to cause photosensitivity include the following: Bitter orange, lemon, cumin, angelica, verbena, opoponax, rue, and lime.

8. **Keep essential oils away from the eyes and never apply them directly to the respiratory tract.** Always wash your hands after working with or applying essential oils to the skin to prevent accidentally smearing your eyes with any irritating essential oils. In case you do accidentally rub essential oils into your eyes, rinse them out immediately under running water. Do not rub your eyes as this could cause the essential oils to penetrate further in.

   Also, do not hold the essential oil container too close to your nose when inhaling the aroma of its contents. The direct application of essential oils onto one's respiratory tracts can irritate them. Essential oils are very concentrated in any case, so you would only need to open a bottle of such to get a whiff. Better yet, invest in an essential oil burner that distributes the scent of the essential oils more evenly in a room to be on the safer side.

Essential oils that can irritate the mucous membrane
include the following: cinnamon, oregano, clove,
spearmint, savory, thyme, and allspice.

9. **Unless you've had a great deal of training in
aromatherapy or are under the guidance of one
who has had such, you should never take
essential oils orally for medicinal reasons.**
Essential oils are so concentrated that a drop of them is
usually the equivalent of about 75 or so cups of tea
brewed from the herb or fruit that they are distilled
from, and are thus toxic, even poisonous, if consumed
improperly. The only time that it is acceptable to ingest
essential oils is when minute amounts (a drop or two) of
them are added to food.

10. **Do not use the same kinds of essential oils
over a prolonged period of time.** This can lead to
the accumulation of certain chemicals in the system
that can be quite toxic, and can also expose the liver and
the kidneys to harmful components in the essential oils
over time. The sole exception to this safety rule is when
the essential oil blend or application is used on the face
as this is a relatively small area of the body. Otherwise,
vary the kinds of essential oils applied so that the body
has ample time to process them and also so you can
benefit from the features offered by other essential oils.
The recommended duration for applying a specific
blend of essential oils on the body is no more than two
weeks. After that, simply switch to another blend.

11. **In case you overexpose yourself to a certain
kind of essential oil, get some fresh air.** This is
particularly advisable if you end up inhaling too much
of an essential oil's aromas (which can lead to
headaches, dizziness, and nausea). In case you suffer

skin irritation from the application of essential oil onto the skin, rub straight vegetable oil onto your skin to dilute the concentration. Do not apply water as this will disperse the said oil further onto your skin.

In the cases of the following essential oils, don't apply them to your skin at all as they are well known irritants: dwarf pine, wintergreen, thyme, pimento, cinnamon, clove, and savory.

12. **If you are pregnant or are above the age of 65, consult a physician prior to using aromatherapy for therapeutic reasons.** The doctor will not only ascertain whether the said treatment method is suitable for you, but will also advise you on which essential oils are suitable for your condition. Some essential oils can produce aromas that are much too potent for pregnant women, and can even induce those who are undergoing particularly sensitive pregnancies to experience a miscarriage. The elderly who are recovering from an operation or suffering from heart disease, on the other hand, should tread especially carefully.

How to Use Essential Oils

Essential oils for aromatherapy can easily be incorporated in anyone's lifestyle. Remember that there are some essential oils with specific usage instructions, but it is still important to perform the initial safety tests. Here are general usage methods for a lot of essential oils:

1. **Direct Inhalation** – Perhaps the easiest way to use essential oils is by direct inhalation. This can be done by adding 3-4 drops of the essential oil on a tissue paper and positioning the paper near your nose. Do not rub or

hold the tissue paper directly on your nose since it may cause irritation.

2. **Steam Inhalation** – Steam inhalations are also proven to be beneficial for nasal conditions such as colds, congestion, and minor headaches. The most common oils used for steam inhalations are *eucalyptus, peppermint,* and *rosemary.* For essential oils, boil 2 cups of water and pour into a bowl. Add about 3-7 drops of the oil into the bowl and position your head about 12 inches away from the bowl. Inhale the steam slowly and maintain your pace. Stop the inhalation immediately if you feel any discomfort or irritation.

3. **Air Freshening** – Aromatherapy essential oils can be used as an air freshener by doing the steam inhalation steps and letting the bowl sit in a room, or by using specific aromatherapy equipment such as a lamp scent ring or a diffuser. Certain essential oils can also be used as effective insect repellants simply by spraying household items.

4. **Massage** – Performing an aromatherapy massage is best done by a qualified practitioner. Usually, the oils used for massage are safely diluted using either soya, olive, grapeseed, or almond oil to avoid adverse reactions. Also make sure to use essential oils appropriate for massage use.

5. **As a bath additive.** This is a great way to enjoy both the inhalation and air freshening benefits of essential oils. Adding a few drops of scented essential oils to a warm bubble bath creates soothing vapors that are suited for inhalation while also giving the oils an avenue for being absorbed directly into the skin.

There are also many other uses for aromatherapy essential oils in your everyday lives. A lot of essential oils can be used for baths, lotions, facial toners, soaps, and other natural products, but it requires the proper knowledge if you wish to create them yourself.

A sample recipe for a simple, lavender-scented lotion is as follows:

Ingredients

1 tablespoon beeswax

5 drops of pure lavender essential oil

1/3 cup coconut oil (virgin coconut oil is said to especially beneficial for the skin)

Procedure

1.) Place the coconut oil and the beeswax in a measuring cup. (Use a measuring cup that is made out of heat-resistant glass or plastic.)

2.) Fill a sturdy-bottomed saucepan or pot halfway with water. Carefully position the measuring cup inside its interior so that the water comes up to half of the measuring cup, and that the measuring cup is not touching the sides of the pot.

3.) Carefully place the saucepan or pot over a stove on medium heat. Stir the coconut oil and beeswax mixture constantly until the mass has melted completely. Remove from heat and set aside. Let the mixture cool until it is no longer too hot to touch.

4.) Once the mixture has cooled, whip it for about three minutes with an electric egg beater. This will introduce air into the mixture and will make it especially fluffy.

5.)   Add in the lavender essential oils and stir vigorously to fully integrate it into the lotion.

6.)   Scoop or spoon into an opaque jar or bottle and store away from heat or direct sunlight. The lotion will retain its scent for about two weeks, so use it up by that time.

Creating Blends

Finally, aromatherapy practitioners can blend together essential oils to achieve a desired effect. Essential oils are blended together for *aromatic effects,* or to achieve a specific fragrance, or for *therapeutic effects,* which heavily emphasizes on the ingredients' therapeutic benefits rather than their scents. The best way to create blends is to use only unadulterated essential oils, and then add carrier oils afterwards.

Essential oil recipes for specific health concerns will be introduced to you in the following chapters.

Chapter 3 – Basic Blending Information

Expert aromatherapy practitioners say: *Aromatherapy is an excellent way to treat various health problems naturally, but it should still not be considered as a substitute for proper medication especially for serious conditions.*

The concept of aromatherapy is understood as the use of natural essential oils to deal with a particular health-related concern by an individual. With this in mind, certain essential oils are known to be effective for remedying emotional problems with the right use.

Thus, prior to starting your blending process, you need to ask yourself a few key questions, which include:

1.) What will the purpose of the blended essential oil mixture be ultimately? The answer to this question will determine the kinds of essential oils you need to use, whether you will need floral ones or citrusy ones (or both).

2.) Will the blend be used via direct inhalation or via direct application onto the skin? This will narrow down the list of essential oils you came up with as a result of the first question, as some essential oils are unsuitable for direct inhalation and/or application onto the skin.

Basic Blending

For the rest of the chapters of this book, you will be introduced to various recipes consisting of different essential oils and the quantity of *drops* to be used for each blend. First, you will need a specific set of requirements for basic blending. For general aromatherapy purposes, here is a list of items you may want to acquire prior to blending:

Aromatherapy & Essential Oil Recipes For Beginners 2nd Edition

1. **Individual Essential Oils** – Of course, you will primarily rely on essential oils to create your blends with. The specific recipes found in this book will provide you with necessary essential oils for each blend. Visit your local aromatherapy store or shop online to acquire these individual essential oils.

2. **Individual Carriers** – Carrier oils are what you dilute your essential oils with. Carrier oils are derived from the *fatty portions* of plants such as the seeds, kernels, and nuts. In the world of aromatherapy, carrier oils are duly named since they *carry* the 100% unadulterated essential oils deemed too harsh to be used on their own. Other carriers can also be used for basic blending such as *natural unscented lotion, pink Himalayan salt,* and *liquid castile soap.*

For some of the recipes in this book, you may be required to use carrier oils for dilution. Although in some cases the carrier oil will be specified, just choose from the following in case only a *carrier oil* is indicated:

Apricot Kernel Oil	*Avocado Oil*
Camellia Seed Oil	*Cranberry Seed Oil*
Fractionated Coconut Oil	*Grapeseed Oil*
Hazelnut Oil	*Hempseed Oil*
Jojoba	*Macadamia Nut Oil*
Meadowfoam Oil	*Olive Oil*
Peanut Oil	*Pecan Oil*
Pomegranate Seed Oil	*Borage Seed Oil*
Evening Primrose Oil	*Sesame Oil*
Sweet Almond Oil	*Sunflower Oil*
Seabuckthorn Berry Oil	*Kukui Nut Oil*
Watermelon Seed Oil	

3. **Jars and Spray bottles** – It is necessary for aromatherapy practitioners to use containers to store unused blends. For general storage, you should use glass bottles with orifice reducers and firm caps. Other container options include glass jars with lids, glass spray bottles, and empty nasal inhalers. You should also opt for glass jars or spray bottles that have opaque colors to protect your essential oil blends from harsh lighting as even such can cause their aromas to evaporate or dissipate. In storing your unused essential oil blends, make sure to put them in a cool, dark place (i.e., nowhere near the window sill).

4. **Mixing Apparatus** – When blending essential oils, it is much preferable to use glassware with a matching glass stir rod so they are easier to clean. It is also recommended to use beakers or measuring cups to make precise measurements. And in case, you will be heating the carrier oils for your essential oil blend, make sure you opt for either heatproof plastic or glass to prevent the container from melting or warping. It should also go without saying that you should rinse out your mixing apparatus after every use to eliminate the risk of cross-contamination. Eventually, should you become serious about the craft and practice of blending essential oils, you might want to invest in glassware (e.g., beakers or measuring cups) that you can allocate for each category (e.g., minty, herbaceous, woodsy, floral, etc.) of essential oils to prevent any scent residue from a previous batch affecting your scent mixture.

5. **Others** – If you are serious about aromatherapy, you may also want to use labels to organize your supply. It is also advisable to use a notebook to maintain a record of your oils and blends. A chart that classifies essential oils according to their aroma and their therapeutic benefits

might also come in handy for the times when you need to whip up an essential oil remedy on the spot.

Additionally, you should know the blending classifications of oils to make blending easier. In essential oil blending, there are **4** classifications: the *personifier,* the *enhancer,* the *equalizer,* and the *modifier.*

The **Personifier** makes up about 1-5% of the blend. These essential oils produce much stronger and longer-lasting aromas backed with substantial therapeutic benefits.

The **Enhancer** makes up about 50-80% of the blend. Although the majority of the blend is composed of the enhancer, the main purpose of enhancers is only to amplify the therapeutic properties of other components in the blend. A characteristic of enhancers is that they do not produce aromas as strong as personifiers.

The **Equalizer** makes up about 10-15% of the blend. It is a vital component that acts as the *bridge* that provides balance for the other essential oils in the blend. The equalizing essential oils also usually possess weaker scents than personifiers.

The **Modifier** makes up about 5-8% of the blend. The modifiers are minor ingredients that add the "finishing touches" to the blend. Just like enhancers and equalizers, modifiers also possess weaker scents than personifiers.

Finally, it is important to note that these blending classifications are only used for creating compound base essential oils, which means these are just generalized instructions if you are to choose to experiment with essential oils and aromas.

Recipes for use in aromatherapy that can be found in the following chapters in this book may not follow the basic classifications exactly, instead, they will be provided with more specific instructions.

Chapter 4 – Emotional Well-being

The ability of essential oils to produce positive effects in a person's emotional state is covered in aromatherapy's psychological effects. The fragrance of essential oils triggers a reaction in the brain, which in turn directly affects a person's emotions.

How to use blends

Blending essential oils in aromatherapy is very simple. It only involves the ingredient essential oils, glassware mixing items, a container, and if required, a carrier oil. For basic blending, simply mix all of the ingredients well on the glassware and store in the container.

In aromatherapy, the blends can be used in multiple ways. Some blends are good only for inhalation applications, while some can be created for use in a *diffuser, bath, massage,* and as an *aerosol.*

First, the *diffuser* used in aromatherapy can be purchased from diffuser manufacturers. If you want to purchase a diffuser, feel free to explore and choose the one of your preference. As long as the diffuser works, the price and the brand do not matter. You can also use *homemade* diffusion methods to achieve the same effect offered by commercial diffusers. The *steam inhalation method* (see Chapter 2) works by releasing the aroma of essential oils into an area; just like a diffuser.

Blends can be used to create bath oils, bath salts, massage oils, and air fresheners. A lot of the blend recipes listed on this book can be used for creating these aromatherapy products. You simply need to adjust the amount of drops to the equivalent drops indicated in the recipe. Just make sure that the ratio of the essential oils in each blend is consistent when trying to reach a specific number of drops.

For example, you are trying to create a *stress relieving bath oil* using 3 drops clary sage oil, 1 drop lemon oil, and 1 drop lavender oil. Since the recipe for creating bath oils is **15 drops** of the blend and 2 ounces of carrier oil, you will then add **9 drops** of clary sage oil, **3 drops** of lemon oil, and **3 drops** of lavender oil for a total of **15 drops.** It is okay to add a little less or more than 15 drops since maintaining the ratio of the blend is far more important than the recipe for the aromatherapy product itself.

With all these in mind, here are the recipes for creating the following aromatherapy products:

1. **Bath Oil** – **15-20** drops of blend, **2** ounces of carrier oil – Store in a glass bottle

2. **Bath Salt** – **15-24** drops of blend, **3** cups salt (*Sea salt, Dead sea salt, Epsom salt,* or *Himalayan pink salt*), and **1** tbsp. of any carrier oil – Store in a glass jar

3. **Massage Oil** – **10-12** drops of blend, **1** ounce carrier oil – Store in a glass bottle

4. **Aerosol** – **1.5** ounces of *hydrosol* or distilled water, **30-40** drops of blend – Store in a clean spray container

Another important item to have in aromatherapy blending is a *dropper bottle top* or a separate *dropper* to make accurate measurements for the recipes.

Finally, remember to use safety precautions before creating or using aromatherapy products (see Chapter 2).

Aromatherapy for Stress Relief

Stress is your body's natural reaction to certain threatening events, also called as stressors. Stress pumps up your body with hormones *adrenaline, cortisol,* and *epinephrine.* These hormones help you react to stressors, but too much stress can cause many physical, emotional, and mental symptoms. When you inhale air that has been scented with the right blend of essential oils (i.e., the ones intended to relieve stress), the olfactory receptors in your nose transmit a signal to the brain's limbic system. The latter, which is in charge of processing our emotions, then reacts to the signal from the aromatherapy by initiating a chemical reaction that tells the brain (and the rest of the body) to relax.

Combating the effects of excessive stress with aromatherapy is one great way to relax without resorting to more toxic or addictive measures like imbibing alcohol or smoking cigarettes. And the best part is, aromatherapy not only helps you melt away the effects of excessive stress momentarily, but it can also stimulate certain neural chemical processes that can fight off infection. This then strengthens the immune system, making you far less vulnerable to illness even when you are under a great deal of stress.

Apart from adding the following aromatherapy blends to warm bubble baths for distressing, you can also have your masseuse or masseur use them (but don't forget to add the carrier oils for protecting your skin, of course) during a massage. This way, you get the triple benefit from a deep tissue massage, the relaxing aroma of an essential oil blend, as well as from the body's absorption of the essential oils. This powerful combination is usually enough to root out even the most stubborn tension points and stress from your body.

Lastly, one of the best things about using essential oils for stress relief is that there are a handful of them that can somehow provide the exact effect that a patient is looking for. Referred to as "adaptogens," these essential oils can individually provide different effects to different people. For instance, an adaptogen sort of essential oil can give a calming effect to a stressed person with heightened feelings of agitation while providing restorative effects to another stressed-out person who might feel burned out and lethargic.

Here are the recipes in aromatherapy that helps relieve stress-related problems:

1. 3 drops *Clary Sage Oil,* 1 drop *Lemon Oil,* and 1 drop *Lavender Oil*

2. 3 drops *Bergamot Oil,* 1 drop *Geranium Oil,* 1 drop *Frankincense Oil*

3. 3 drops *Grapefruit Oil,* 1 drop *Jasmine Oil,* and 1 drop *Ylang Ylang Oil*

4. 3 drops *Lemon Oil,* 2 drops *Rosemary Oil,* 1 drop *Basil Oil*

Storage: Glass bottle (Firm/dropper cap)
Mixture: Add all ingredients and mix well for about 1-2 minutes

The aforementioned recipes can be used either in a massage, in home aromatherapy diffuser kits, or in warm bubble baths. Whichever option you choose, you might want to try an assortment of essential oil blends to determine which one meets your stress relief needs best without overpowering your senses. Do tread carefully when measuring out the amount of essential oil blends for your massage, diffuser, and/or bubble bath so that you don't risk an attack of dizziness or nausea from using too much of the essential oil. As with many concentrated substances, a little goes a long, long way.

Should you want to try your hand at making your own essential oil blend for combating stress relief, here is a list of other essential oils you can try mixing, apart from the ones mentioned in the recipes above:

1.) Orange blossom oil. This essential oil is distilled from neroli blossoms, and is prized for its calming qualities. The aroma of orange blossom oil is also said to encourage feelings of hopefulness, confidence, and peace, sentiments that any stressed-out person would be grateful for.

2.) Orange oil. One of the most popular citrus essential oils, orange oil is used in many essential oil blends for its uplifting effect. A study from a Japanese university was even able to deduce that patients who benefited from aromatherapy sessions where orange oil figured prominently not only cut their antidepressant dosage significantly, but also ended up normalizing both their endocrine and immune system.

3.) Rose oil. This floral essential oil both revitalizes a tired mind and promotes a general sense of well-being. However, since this is among the most concentrated of the essential oils, the pure kind is rather overpowering, so mix it into a blend instead of using it on its own. And even when it has been incorporated into an essential oil blend, it should be used in tiny amounts (i.e., a dab or two) for optimum effect.

Aromatherapy for Happiness and Relaxation

Aromatherapy is popular for achieving sensations of bliss, peacefulness, and calmness. *Orange Oil* is an excellent start to be used unadulterated to provide quick positive feelings and emotional wellness, as citrus oils are particularly prized by aromatherapy experts for being the most uplifting.

However, it is still better to use a combination to provide the best effect, and to balance out the sharpness of the acidity that can sometimes accompany citrus-based essential oils.

Vanilla essential oils, for instance, can also be mixed with citrus-based essential oils to produce a blend that can encourage feelings of happiness and relaxation. Citrus essential oils uplift the mind and the spirit, while the scent of vanilla often conjures up memories of a childhood birthday cake and can thus help one revisit happier, less complicated times.

Lavender essential oils are also at the top of the list when it comes to stimulating a relaxing effect. Medical journals that focus on the health benefits of aromatherapy often cite it as an essential oil that significantly lowers heightened heart rates, skin temperatures, and blood pressure, all indicators of a tense patient on edge.

Here are some of the basic essential oil blends and recipes to help you achieve a state of emotional bliss:

1. 2 drops *Orange Oil,* 2 drops *Grapefruit Oil,* and 1 drop *Ylang Ylang* or *Rose Oil*

2. 3 drops *Bergamot Oil,* 1 drop *Ylang Ylang Oil,* and 1 drop *Grapefruit Oil*

3. 2 drops *Bergamot Oil,* 2 drops *Sandalwood Oil,* 1 drop *Clove Oil,* and 1 drop *Ylang Ylang Oil*

4. 2 drops *Orange Oil,* 2 drops *Frankincense Oil,* and 1 drop *Geranium Oil*

Storage: Glass bottle (Firm/dropper cap)
Mixture: Add all ingredients and mix well for about 1-2 minutes

Apart from the essential oils mentioned above, you can also try making your own essential oil blend by choosing from among the following essential oils below:

1.) Marjoram oil. This essential oil is favored for its ability to relieve inflammation and to relax the muscles, as well as to promote a more restful sleep. The ancient Greeks also referred to it as the "joy of the mountains" while the ancient Romans revered it as the "herb of happiness" for its uplifting effects. Marjoram essential oils work best as equalizers or enhancers in the blending process.

2.) Cedarwood oil. The Native Americans were on to something when they used cedarwood in their rituals to commune with the spirits as its fumes stimulate the limbic center of the brain as well as the production of melatonin in the pineal glands. Melatonin is a hormone that helps the body relax and regulate its sleeping cycles.

Aromatherapy for Anger Management

Anger is a very powerful negative emotion that may result in actions and poor decisions that a person may regret afterwards. Essential oils help prevent an individual from giving in to the impulses that anger can bring by opening up the mind and helping him or her to process the situation differently. Some essential oil blends have also been known to help balance one's emotions better, leading to a clearer head.

While it may not always be possible to indulge in an aromatherapy breathing session whenever one is struck by feelings of bubbling rage (especially since these commonly occur in the workplace), it is advised that one affected by such should step away from the situation a bit and take some deep breaths to calm down. Having a bottle of hand wash or hand lotion scented with the essential oil blends meant for alleviating intense anger readily accessible in one's work place can also help the process greatly. Even the simple act of washing your hands with the scented hand wash or soap while taking deep, reassuring breaths can really do wonders for dispelling your anger and help you take control of such incendiary emotions better.

Feelings of anger may not occur to you every day, but whenever you feel like you need to alleviate your anger for whatever reason, try the following recipes:

1. 3 drops *Orange Oil*, 1 drop *Vetiver Oil*, and 1 drop *Rose Oil*

2. 3 drops *Orange Oil*, and 2 drops *Patchouli Oil*

3. 2 drops *Orange Oil*, 2 drops *Bergamot Oil*, and 1 drop *Roman Chamomile Oil*

4. 3 drops *Bergamot Oil*, 1 drop *Ylang Ylang Oil*, and 1 drop *Jasmine Oil*

Storage: Glass bottle (Firm/dropper cap)
Mixture: Add all ingredients and mix well for about 1-2 minutes

Other essential oils that you can mix together for your own unique anger management blend include the following:

1.) Geranium oil. Geranium oil's calming effects are not only good for inducing sleep, but they are also capable of leading a person to release festering negative emotions, which in turn, can dispel most of a person's flared-up anger. Rubbing a couple of drops of the concentrated form of Geranium oil into one's temples or onto one's nape helps greatly when one is trying to keep a handle on one's emotions in front of a difficult situation.

2.) German Chamomile. Much like Roman Chamomile oil, German Chamomile oil can also dispel anger when taken in via steam inhalation. Use it as a potent personifier in your custom essential oil blend, and benefit from its ability to bring clarity to your mind as well as a much-needed stability for volatile emotions.

Aromatherapy for Healthy Sleep

An underlying problem that may contribute in a person's stress and unstable emotions is the unhealthy sleeping habits. Given that the 21st century is host to an increasingly fast-paced lifestyle accompanied by the glaring screens of tablets, laptops, and smart phones, patients who wish to regulate their sleeping patterns for the better can benefit from key essential oil blends that seek to offset the sleep-deterring effects of the previously-mentioned technology.

Aromatherapy induces better sleep quality in a variety of ways. Some essential oils calm a frantic mind to pave the way for restful slumber while a few specialize in lowering blood pressure and heart rate to reduce the body's tension.

Apart from the basic methods of introducing essential oils or blends into the body via direct inhalation, aromatherapy also works best as a sleep aid when combined with other practices such as deep-tissue massages. The latter is particularly effective at bringing about better sleep quality as it can also relieve pain and unknot tense muscles, which helps the body relax further into sleep. Essential oils or blends rubbed into the body during the massage will also help them penetrate deeper into the body, and render them more effective. The aromas given off by the essential oil blends during the massage could also help clear the patient's olfactory and respiratory tracts, encouraging better, deeper breathing, a quality that is central to good sleep quality.

The basic rule of a good sleep is to get 7-9 hours of quality sleep at night. But given the modern lifestyle of an average person today, this is nearly impossible to do. Fortunately, aromatherapy has an answer for this problem. Just follow this recipe for a sleep-inducing blend:

1. 2 drops *Roman Chamomile Oil*, 1 drop *Clary Sage Oil*, and 1 drop *Bergamot Oil*

2. 3 drops *Chamomile Oil*, 3 drops *Sandalwood Oil*, 2 drops *Lavender Oil*, and 2 drops *Ylang Ylang Oil*

Tip: For better sleep, you can add about 1-2 drops of the blend to a tissue and place it under your pillow.

Storage: Glass bottle (Firm/dropper cap)
Mixture: Add all ingredients and mix well for about 1-2 minutes

Other essential oils that can also be used to make your own sleep-inducing essential oil blend include the following:

1.) Valerian oil. While Valerian oil is sometimes used as a stimulant, it also does wonders for reducing anxiety. After being mixed with other essential oils like chamomile or lavender and with a suitable carrier oil, Valerian oil is best applied or massaged onto the wrists or on the soles of the feet for better penetration into the body.

2.) Cedarwood oil. Cedarwood oil can also be used in essential oil blends for improving sleep as it helps to regulate one's sleep cycle. Patients who are recovering from jet lag or those who work graveyard shifts can largely benefit from the regulating effects that cedarwood oil can have on their irregular sleeping patterns. Inhaling or massaging an essential oil blend that contains cedarwood oil can also rest one's internal body clock.

Chapter 5 – Skin and Hair Care

Long before people would debate over whether a certain kind
of shampoo or facial wash had parabens or not, essential oils
were already being used as a key component of many natural
cosmetics and beauty aids. Since essential oils, by nature,
contain what is referred to as the life force of potent plants
and flowers, their use was thought to transfer some of the
said plants and flowers' more desirable characteristics onto
the skin and hair of the patient.

Furthermore, essential oils were also the world's first multi-
tasking cosmetics as they served as medicine, perfume, and
beauty aids simultaneously. After all, essential oils were
initially developed to address certain health concerns like
skin irritations (e.g., acne or dry scalp), regulate bodily
functions, and flush out toxins or wastes from the body. And
the result of all these objectives being achieved was the
enhancement and preservation of one's natural beauty, given
that such could not be achieved without looking like the
poster child for glowing health.

While advances in science and technology may have resulted
in some of the most up-to-date and top of the line beauty
aids and treatments, skin and hair care products with an
essential oil base remain as relevant as ever. This is primarily
because they are produced without any synthetic ingredients
or harmful chemicals that are often hidden in mass-
produced beauty products. Making your own essential oil
beauty aids also presents the added benefit of knowing
exactly what goes into the products that you use on your
body, as well the level of control that you can exert over the
selection of such.

Aromatherapy & Essential Oil Recipes For Beginners 2nd Edition

The use of natural essential oils in aromatherapy is proven to be effective for physical health concerns, including skin and hair care. To accomplish this, you will need to follow these recipes and blends for specific concerns in your health.

General Facial Toner

Your skin not only protects your internal organs from external elements, it is also the part of *you* that you present to the world. This is why anyone should know the importance of keeping their skin healthy from the inside out. For this effect, you can try this recipe of blended essential oils for use as an everyday toner:

10 drops of *Grapefruit Oil,* 5 drops of *Tea Tree Oil,* 5 drops of *Cypress Oil,* 3 oz. of *Witch Hazel Hydrosol,* and 1 oz. *High-Proof Vodka*

Storage: Glass bottle (Firm/dropper cap)
Mixture: Add all ingredients and mix well for about 1-2 minutes

Important: Shake the recipe well before each use, and make sure to perform the essential safety precautions before applying any aromatherapy product on your skin.

Facial Toner for Combination Skin

Combination skin is comprised of both dry and oily skin. Since the T-zone (the part of the face that's composed of the forehead, eyebrows, and nose) is oily, and the U-zone (the cheeks and the chin) is dry, using two kinds of toners is sometimes necessary. The following recipe, however, is good for balancing both zones of combination skin.

1 drop of *Patchouli Oil,* 1 drop of *Palmarosa Oil,* 7 drops of *Lavender Oil,* 1 drop *Ylang Ylang Oil,* 1 drop *Rose Geranium oil,* 250 ml *Lavender Hydrosol.*

Storage: Glass bottle (Firm/dropper cap)
Mixture: Add all ingredients and mix well for about 1-2 minutes

Facial Toner for Sensitive Skin

Sensitive skin is normally averse to harsh treatments or chemicals. Thus, there are no citrus oils in their facial toner recipe since they have a tendency to increase the skin's photosensitivity or its aversion to light. Apart from being very gentle, this facial toner recipe also has a calming effect on inflamed or irritated skin. This toner can also be used for those with mature, aging skin.

3 drops of *Frankincense oil*, 1 drop *Chamomile oil*, 3 drops *Lavender oil*, 250 ml *Rose water*, 3 drops *Sandalwood oil*, 5 ml *Glycerin*

Storage: Glass bottle (Firm/dropper cap)
Mixture: Add all ingredients and mix well for about 1-2 minutes

Acne

Everyone in this world will experience mild to severe acne at some point in their lives. Acne forms due to blockages on pores where dirt, oil, and bacteria thrive. It usually occurs during the adolescent years, but some may experience acne even during adulthood.

Treating acne using aromatherapy will produce natural results by fighting bacteria, cleansing the skin, reducing inflammation, and reducing pigmentation from healing pimples. To do this, use the following recipe:

6 drops of *Lavender Oil*, 5 drops of *Tea Tree Oil (or Manuka Oil)*, 1 drop *Geranium Oil*, and 1 oz. of *Jojoba* or *Fractionated Coconut Carrier Oil*

Storage: Glass bottle (Firm/dropper cap)
Mixture: Add all ingredients and mix well for about 1-2 minutes

You can also make a facial toner for oily or acne-prone skin by using the following recipe:

3 drops *Tea Tree oil*, 3 drops *Petitgrain oil*, 1 drop *Rose Geranium oil*, 3 drops *Palmarosa oil*, 3 drops *Lemongrass oil*, 250 ml *Witch Hazel Hydrosol*

Storage: Glass bottle (Firm/dropper cap)
Mixture: Add all ingredients and mix well for about 1-2 minutes

Peppermint Sugar Body Scrub

Prior to moisturizing with lotion, it's best to remove dead cells from the skin's surface by exfoliating. The following recipe incorporates peppermint essential oil and grapefruit essential oil to soothe tired, dry skin and to invigorate your senses in the shower, respectively. For best results, use this body scrub recipe in the shower at least twice a week. Follow through with any of the succeeding body lotion recipes to lock in the moisture.

250 grams *Coarse Brown Sugar*, 60 ml *Sweet Almond Oil*, 10 drops *Peppermint Oil*, 10 ml *Glycerin*, 15 drops *Grapefruit Oil*, the zest of half a *Grapefruit*

Storage: Glass Jar with a tightly sealed cap

Mixture: Combine the sugar with the sweet almond oil, glycerin, and the grapefruit zest until they are well-mixed. Gradually add the drops of peppermint and grapefruit essential oils, combining well after each addition.

Aromatherapy Skin Lotion

To help protect your skin and keep it moisturized during the day, you can try applying your very own skin lotion made entirely out of natural essential oils. To do this, simply follow this recipe:

20 drops of *Sandalwood Oil,* 10 drops of *Patchouli Oil,* 5 drops of *Carrot Seed Oil,* and 8 oz. *unscented natural lotion base*

Storage: Glass bottle (Firm cap, use a funnel to store lotion)
Mixture: Add all ingredients and mix well for about 1-2 minutes

Aromatherapy Hair Shampoo

Washing your hair with natural essential oils effectively removes accumulated dirt while keeping your hair healthy and smelling great. For creating your own aromatherapy shampoo using essential oils, you will need about 7 oz. of unscented shampoo base for the recipe. This can be purchased individually from natural products and aromatherapy shops.

To create your own aromatherapy shampoo, use the following recipe:

40 drops of *Lavender Oil,* 10 drops of *Rosemary Oil,* 5 drops of *Ylang Ylang Oil,* and about 1 tbsp. of *Jojoba Oil*

Storage: Glass bottle (Firm/dropper cap)
Mixture: Add all ingredients and mix well for about 1-2 minutes

Hair Conditioner

After washing, you can apply a hair conditioner to further protect your hair from damage. To do this, follow this simple recipe (for one application only):

1-3 drops of *Rosemary Oil,* and 1 tbsp. *Jojoba Carrier Oil*

For this recipe, simply mix the oils in a small bowl and apply evenly on your hair. Let the conditioner sit on your hair for about 15-30 minutes and then rinse off.

Chapter 6 – Aromatherapy for Weight Loss

Aromatherapy works for people trying to lose weight by triggering brain reactions that mimics the sensation of being full to control cravings. This mechanism will effectively inhibit the urge to eat more food, and will therefore enable any individual to achieve his or her target weight by eating less. And since essential oils are also quite adept at regulating moods or uplifting despondency, the emotional reasons behind a person's tendency to overeat (e.g., to comfort himself or herself) are further eliminated.

Further studies even suggest that the fragrance of certain essential oils actually helps the body to *burn fat*. Of course, there is still much debate about the alleged scientific evidence claiming such, but scientists were able to determine that aromatherapy had an effect on women's weight during a 6-week experiment in *Wonkwang Health Science College* in Korea.

However, it should be noted that aromatherapy is not a silver bullet for effective weight loss. Simply inhaling a special blend of essential oils will not shed off unwanted pounds, unless the practice is accompanied with a proper diet and effective exercise. What aromatherapy simply does is to make the process a bit easier by limiting hunger pangs and keeping the mind focused on the goal. In a nutshell, aromatherapy is but a complementary course of action for a comprehensive weight loss plan that should include other measures.

Essential Oils to Control Hunger

To help control the amount of food you eat, you can use the following essential oils for direct inhalation:

Peppermint Oil – This essential oil is proven to relieve digestive problems as well as to promote healthy digestion. On an emotional level, peppermint essential oils are a good alternative to indulging in calorie-laden sweets or pastries. Rather than gorging one's self on such, the patient can simply pour a few drops of peppermint oil on a handkerchief and inhale the scent deeply so that she or he can experience a sense of relief in the face of a stressful scenario.

Orange Oil – The powerful emotional enhancing effects of orange oil helps build self-control and willpower required to control your diet. And since orange oil also figures prominently in essential oil blends that are meant to forge feelings of happiness and optimism, it can also help users to overcome the effects of depression, some of which include overeating.

Grapefruit Oil – The scent of grapefruit oil is known to control urges to eat and helps metabolism. Its cheery scent is also prized for relieving stress, which is one of the main causes of overeating. Applied to a body scrub, grapefruit oil releases enzymes that help break down layers of cellulite.

Bergamot Oil – This essential oil has stress-relieving and calming effects which are incredibly helpful for suppressing hunger. Bergamot oil is also advisable for people who "stress eat," or those who tend to binge when under a great deal of pressure and tension. The scent of bergamot oil is said to encourage the endocrine system to release hormones that calm the mind and body, thus steering it away from "stress eating" episodes.

Ginger Oil – Like peppermint oil, ginger oil also helps the body digest the food better so that there are less sugars or carbohydrates left behind that turn into fat. A whiff of ginger oil is also known to boost energy levels, making it much easier for someone on a weight loss regimen to get through a rigorous exercise routine.

Cinnamon Oil- Excellent for detoxing the body and for improving one's digestion processes and circulation, cinnamon oil via direct inhalation also helps foster positive body images, which are far more encouraging to those who wish to lose weight successfully.

Essential Oils Weight Loss Pills

If you want to take essential oils a little further in achieving results for weight loss, you might want to try creating your own weight loss pills made of essential oils. For this recipe, you will need *empty gelatin pill capsules* (0 size or 500 mg capsules).

For this method, use 4 drops of *Lemon Oil,* 4 drops of *Peppermint Oil,* and *Grapeseed Oil* as your carrier. Simply add the essential oils and fill the rest of the capsule with the Grapeseed Oil using the dropper. Take twice a day.

Note: Make sure to perform an allergy test on your skin before ingesting essential oils.

Citrus Essential Oils Weight Loss Smelling Salts

In case you're wary of ingesting essential oils (as they are quite concentrated); you can use the following recipe for smelling salts instead. Store these in a metal or opaque glass receptacle with a filter to keep the salts in, and take a whiff whenever you feel the need to control or suppress the appetite.

4 drops *Orange Oil*, 1 drop *Sandalwood Oil*, 30 drops *Grapefruit Oil*, 10 g *Coarse Sea Salt*

Storage: Small Metal or Opaque Glass Receptacle with Filter (If you have such a container that can be worn around the neck or on a chain, it would be so much better.)

Mixture: Combine the essential oils together, and then add in the salt. Stir the mixture until the salt has absorbed all the essential oils, and then transfer to your container of choice.

Chapter 7 – Aromatherapy for Sun Protection

Since it's been established that frequent and unprotected exposure to the sun is the number one cause of accelerated skin aging, it's been a must to apply sunblock before leaving the house. Furthermore, it's been discovered that protective sun care is also needed for the lips apart from the body's overall skin.

In this chapter, some of the moisturizers with essential oils are given a special addition of zinc oxide, a compound that protects the skin from the sun's harmful rays.

Sandalwood Sunblock Lotion

In case you weren't able to grab a bottle of sunblock at the store or if you're wary of the potentially toxic ingredients that may be contained in every bottle of industrially-produced sunblock lotion on the market, you can make your own blend using the following recipe. Sandalwood oil is called for here, but you can also use your favorite essential oil scent.

25 drops *Sandalwood Oil*, 10 drops *Myrrh Oil*, 2 drops *Vetiver Oil*, 10 drops *Carrot Seed Oil*, 2 ounces *Virgin Coconut Oil*, 2 ounces *Shea Butter*, 1 ounce *Cocoa Butter*, 2 ounces *Avocado Oil*, 2 ounces *Beeswax*, 5 grams *Zinc Oxide Powder*

Storage: 4 oz. opaque glass jars

Mixture: In a heatproof glass or plastic measuring cup, combine the two kinds of butters with the beeswax and the virgin coconut oil. Fill a heavy-bottomed pot halfway with water, then carefully place the measuring cup inside it, making sure that it doesn't touch the sides of the pot. Place on a stove that's been set to medium heat, and stir the mixture in the measuring pot constantly until the beeswax has completely melted and you get a smooth, shiny mass that's free of any lumps. Remove from heat and quickly mix in the zinc oxide powder until it's completely dissolved in the mixture. Set the mixture aside until it's lukewarm to the touch, and then stir in the avocado oil and the essential oils. Apply at least twice a day, or every forty-five minutes in case of constant sun exposure.

Peppermint Lip Balm

The skin on our lips is very thin, and is thus even more susceptible to moisture loss and dehydration, as well as to sun damage. This homemade lip balm recipe is not only easy to make, but the addition of peppermint essential oils to the base mixtures provides a nice, cooling effect on the lips that will encourage you to keep applying this throughout the day.

20 g *White Beeswax Beads*, 45 g *Sunflower Oil*, 4 *Vitamin E Oil Tablets*, 20 g *Cocoa Butter*, 12 drops *Peppermint Oil*, 2 drops *Basil Oil*, 2 grams *Zinc Oxide*

Storage: Plastic lip balm tubes or tins

Mixture: In a heatproof glass or plastic measuring cup, combine the beeswax with the sunflower oil and cocoa butter. Break open the Vitamin E oil tablets and empty their contents into the measuring cup. Fill a heavy-bottomed pot halfway with water, then carefully place the measuring cup inside it, making sure that it doesn't touch the sides of the pot. Place on a stove that's been set to medium heat, and stir the mixture in the measuring pot constantly until the beeswax has completely melted and you get a smooth, shiny mass that's free of any lumps. Remove from heat and quickly mix in the zinc oxide until it's dissolved. Set aside until the mixture is merely warm to the touch. Quickly stir in the essential oils, and then pour into your receptacle of choice.

Chapter 8 – Aromatherapy as an Aphrodisiac

A healthy love life and libido is always a sign of good health, but for those who feel that they might need a boost in this department, aromatherapy can provide some much-needed assistance.

The scents of certain essential oils can mimic the effects of arousal by encouraging the flow of blood to certain parts of the body, such as the lips or the skin. In this way, the mind is tricked into an amorous mood, and the rest of the body usually follows suit.

The use of key aromatherapy oils can also create a more relaxed, but also far more sensual atmosphere that's far more conducive to the act of love. Warm scents like cinnamon, for instance, can induce a more passionate mood between two people.

The best way to use aromatherapy as an aphrodisiac is via direct inhalation, thus a few of the essential oils that you can apply to an oil burner to achieve such an effect are as follows:

1.) Neroli or orange blossom essential oil. This is one of the few essential oils out there that has a completely balanced fragrance on its own. Neroli essential oil has a heavy, heady, and intoxicating scent that can both calm nerves (ideal for nervous lovers) and encourage thoughts of romance.

2.) Patchouli essential oil. This essential oil is known for its distinctive earthy aroma that resembles that of incense. Most people also associate it with the free love movement of the 60's and that in itself can encourage an amatory ambience.

3.)   Ylang-ylang oil essential oil. Ylang-ylang flowers have long been prized in Southeast Asia for their sweet, floral aroma that's been known to incite passion between married couples. As an added bonus, ylang-ylang essential oil has also been applied in massages to help impotent lovers overcome their sexual impediments

4.)   Rose essential oil. While this floral essential oil can be rather cloying in big amounts, a few drops of it in massage oil or in a warm bath can result in you or your partner getting second wind for more passionate embraces after a long day at work.

5.)   Sandalwood essential oil. Though the scent of sandalwood can sometimes be present in religious institutions, its woody balsamic aroma has also been prized for its ability to incite passion. As with rose oil, a few drops of pure sandalwood oil in a hot bath or in a massage can go a long way towards creating a sensual and romantic encounter.

Chapter 9 – Essential Oils Categories

Should you wish to make your own essential oil blends, below is a list of the nine distinct categories of essential oils based on their individual scents. Some of them are potent enough on their own, while others are used to balance out a certain blend.

1.) Oriental. These are rich and slightly cloying scents traditionally associated with the East. Essential oils that fall under this category include patchouli, sandalwood, and ginger oils.

2.) Earthy. These essential oils smell of soil and grass, and add a hint of rusticity to any essential oil mixture. Examples of earthy essential oils are those imbued with the essences of vetiver and oak moss.

3.) Minty. These types of essential oils are traditionally prescribed for headaches or for stress relief. Applied directly to the skin, they can give off a cooling effect. Spearmint and peppermint essential oils fall under this category.

4.) Spicy. Essential oils that fall under this category include clove, cinnamon, and nutmeg. They are often used to establish a warm, comforting mood when used in aromatherapy, and can be blended with floral, citrus, or oriental oils to enhance the effect.

5.) Citrus. Citrus-scented or based essential oils are known for their uplifting effects on one's mental well-being, and are commonly invoked by patients who wish to increase their focus or to lift their mood. Lemon, lime, orange, and bergamot oils are some of the most popular citrus essential oils. Out of all the essential oil categories, however, citrus oils are the ones that dissipate the fastest, so you should use them up within one year or less. Thus, unless you plan on using a lot of essential oil blends that call for citrus oil, it would be best to purchase citrus oils in smaller quantities.

6.) Medicinal. These are usually applied directly onto the skin rather than inhaled directly, and are thus mixed into lotions or facial wash. Essential oils like eucalyptus are applied to soothe tired, aching muscles. And with its antibacterial and anti-viral properties, tea tree oil is prescribed for skin pustules, acne, and mild eczema.

7.) Herbaceous. As its name suggests, herbaceous essential oils are derived from kitchen herbs like rosemary, basil, marjoram, or basil. Herbaceous essential oils commonly used to bring about mental clarity, although they can also be inhaled via steam inhalation to clear the respiratory tract or mucous membrane.

8.) Woodsy. Essential oils that fall under this category are derived from the trunks of aromatic trees like cedar or pine. Since they are compatible with all the essential oil categories, woodsy essential oils are used to balance the fragrance composition of any essential oil blend. Essential oils made from aromatic trees with thick resin such as frankincense also last the longest out of all the essential oil categories, and their scents also tend to get richer and more mellow with age.

9.) Floral. Derived from blossoms, floral essential oils like jasmine or neroli are popular choices for perfume or cologne bases, but they also have medicinal value. Lavender essential oil, for instance, is not only good for inducing sleep (as well as improving its overall quality), but also for sanitizing burns.

Conclusion

Thank you again for purchasing this book!

I hope this book was able to help you to gain valuable knowledge and learn specific steps in creating basic essential oil blends.

The next step is to keep on learning about the potential of aromatherapy and essential oils using various sources available to you.

Finally, if you enjoyed this book, please take the time to share your thoughts and post a review on Amazon. We do our best to reach out to readers and provide the best value we can. Your positive review will help us achieve that. It'd be greatly appreciated!

Thank you and good luck!